MINDFULNESS
BREATHE IN - BREATHE OUT

IVANA STRASKA SZAKAL

 England

Mindfulness - Breathe In Breathe Out

All rights reserved. No parts of this book may be reproduced, scanned or distributed in any printed or electronic form without the written permission of the author. Please do not participate in or encourage piracy of copyrighted material in violation of author's rights. Purchase only authorized edition.

Neither the author nor the publisher is engaged in rendering professional advice or service to the individual reader. Information in this book is intended to educate and is not to substitute consulting with medical professionals. All matters regarding your health require medical supervision. Neither the author nor the publisher shall be liable or responsible for any loss or damage allegedly arising from any information or suggestion in this book.

First edition

ISBN 978-1-9998266-2-8

Graphic design by Christopher Gill

Copyright © 2017 by Ivana Straska Szakal

Published by IVANA INTERNATIONAL, England

WHY DO WE NEED THIS BOOK?

This short book is intended to provide a quick step by step guide to get started with mindfulness. The free downloadable audio tracks will assist in establishing a routine and understanding. There are of course many extensive reference books on the market thoroughly explaining what is to know about mindfulness. The uniqueness of this book is to allow anyone who wishes to try mindfulness to do it with economy of time. These chapters intend to simply guide the user do develop basic understanding and a routine. Just to learn and practice.

It should be emphasised that this is a guide to help towards improved well-being it is not intended for those with major issues who should seek medical advice. The explanations in this book are kept brief and provide only the essential information. It explains why we are doing certain things and what we hope to achieve but in the simplest terms possible. There is more information provided at the end the book should you wish skip there. But for now if you wish to get started read here.

TABLE OF CONTENTS

PART ONE
THE BEGINNING

1.	**Understanding**	2
	1.1. Is this the Right Time?	2
	1.2. What Is Mindfulness?	3
	1.3. Why Should We Cultivate Mindfulness?	4
	1.3.1. Mindfulness Has Many Benefits	4
	1.4. Does Science Support Mindfulness?	5
2.	**Mindfulness Through Meditation**	6
	2.1. How To Progress	6
	2.1.1. Ability to Relax	7
	2.1.2. Practise Patience	7
	2.2. Set the Routine	8
	2.3. Place	9
	2.4. How to Start	10
	2.4.1. General Rules	11
	2.4.2. A Few Tips to Advance	12

PART TWO
MINDFULNESS IN STAGES

3.	**Curiosity**	14
	3.1. Aspects of Mindfulness	14
	3.2. Why is Curiosity Important?	14
	3.3. What To Do	15
	3.4. How To Do It	15
	3.5. Examples How to Enhance Curiosity	16
4.	**Awareness**	17
	4.1. Why Do We Increase Awareness?	17
	4.2. What To Do	18
	4.3. How To Do It	19
5.	**Acceptance**	20
	5.1. Why Do We Exercise Acceptance?	20
	5.2. What To Do	21

	5.3. How To Do It	22
6.	**Focus**	**23**
	6.1. Why Do We Change Focus?	23
	6.2. What To Do	24
	6.3. How To Do It	25
7.	**Communication**	**26**
	7.1. What Is Mindful Communication?	26
	7.2. What To Do	27
	7.3. How To Do It	27
8.	**Compassion**	**29**
	8.1. Why Do We Learn Compassion?	29
	8.2. What To Do?	30
	8.3. How To Do It	30
9.	**Kindness**	**32**
	9.1. Why Kindness?	32
	9.2. What to Do	33
	9.3. How To Do It	33

PART THREE
IN SUMMARY

10.	**Living Mindfully**	35

About the Author	36
Resources	37

MINDFULNESS - BREATHE IN BREATHE OUT

PART ONE
THE BEGINNING

CHAPTER 1
understanding

1.1. Is This the Right Time

Despite its long tradition and history mindfulness has become a wanted aspect of modern life. The world's leaders and luminaries are becoming more open about their experiences with mindfulness. Successful entrepreneurs such as Arianna Huffington, Oprah Winfrey, or Ray Dalio reveal how mindfulness helps them to maintain their success and health. Recently more actors and musicians publicly share their experience with mindfulness. Even the great baseball player Michael Jordan hired his own mindfulness coach. Perhaps, we also should give it a try and allow this inspiration to improve our life experience.

Mindfulness is believed to have originated in Buddhism but is now a secular practice undertaken by an increasing number of people as part of their daily routine. Mindfulness can be applied in an entirely practical way. In recent months there has been significant interest in mindfulness as a practical and effective method of making our, often frantic, life less stressful. It can help to improve sleep, cope with challenges, increase control over life and generally makes us feel better.

There have been references on several health related UK television programmes, plus the UK government Schools Minister expressed interest in promoting mindfulness in schools. It has since been introduced into some UK classrooms with over 5,000 teachers trained to teach mindfulness and it has been adopted in some universities as a way of helping students combat stress. Hopefully, the young generation will grow mindful. So, shouldn't we adults give a chance to mindfulness?

We all experience a roller-coaster life with stress, abrupt challenges and losses. The application of mindfulness can help us develop a new approach even if we don't suffer difficult to manage conditions. Most of us do not need to remedy some deep, disabling conditions. We simply wish to feel better about ourselves and life as a whole. We want to enjoy the days as they pass and we wish, hopefully, to age healthy and happy. We long for positive experience with some degree of effective balance and wisdom. We want to develop our full potential to bring value and beauty into our lives. Mindfulness is an amazing and proven tool in aiding us to achieve all these goals. There is no better time to start then now.

1.2. What Is Mindfulness

To understand the principles of mindfulness and to develop the basic skills is not as hard as it may sound. Actually, mindfulness is nothing exotic or new. We all have the ability to be mindful but we don't cultivate it, so we lose it. We have inherent capacities passed down through the centuries from our ancestor who needed to be mindful in a moment to survive.

In essence, mindfulness is paying full attention to the moment and being aware; being engaged with what we are doing in each moment. Mindfulness is to be present and alert as a child would be. It is easy in our hectic modern lives to miss contact with or stop noticing the world around us. We often fail to notice the reality of the way our body feels. We can end up living in our own thoughts without realising how they affect our emotions and behaviour. Mindfulness is about paying attention to the world around us and to our own thoughts and feelings.

There are instants when we are mindful without realizing it. In fact, any time we have moments of being truly aware and present, we are practising mindfulness. We mindfully do activities we love doing, when we forget about time and we are single focused. Hobbies might be a good example of activity we do mindfully and with engagement of the senses. We can think of daydreaming as the opposite of mindfulness. That is the time when we mentally travel and think about the past or future.

To be mindful we don't have to change who we are. We change only our focus. When we cultivate this with simple practice we benefit in many ways. We can formally practise mindfulness as meditation or less formally we can exercise mindfulness within other activities such as walking, eating, talking, breathing, driving, or any other ordinary activity. We can even exercise this informal mindfulness while, for example, brushing teeth or other mundane routines.

1.3. Why Should We Cultivate Mindfulness?

Cultivation of mindfulness enables us to see our current experience more clearly through an awareness of our thoughts and feelings. In this way mindfulness fosters an internal strength helping us to face and cope with day to day pressure and emotionally distressing circumstances or occurrences. It can actively change our lives and our self-perception.

1.3.1. Mindfulness Has Many Benefits

The greatest benefits of mindfulness might be slightly technical but we should be aware that when practicing mindfulness we hugely help ourselves. Recent studies have shown that simple mindfulness actually causes measurable changes in brain activity. We stimulate certain parts of the brain to experience pleasure. This effect can last hours or days. With regular practice the adaptability of the brain allows long-lasting change; its "pathways" or "wiring" changes. In other words the biological structure of our brains can actually change to produce a better attitude with improved positive, productive thinking.

Mindfulness has the potential to allow us to control how much we engage with pleasant or unpleasant thoughts and emotions. It allows the development of emotional flexibility and open mindedness. In essence mindfulness teaches us to:

- experience the present moment.
- pay attention on purpose and meaning.
- focus on both inside and outside ourselves.
- let go of negative thoughts and develop a less judgemental stance.

Mindfulness practise helps us to learn how to let thoughts come and go, not to hold onto them. With mindfulness we deepen the connection with ourselves and our body. Mindfulness develops the ability to take a note of what's happening, to recognize and to be aware. The important relaxing impact consequently improves our performance. We work and study more effectively, remember more, fully attend and pay attention, and overall we expand positive experience.

1.4. Does Science Support Mindfulness?

Within the past few decades, there has been a surge of scientific interest in the investigation of mindfulness both in its psychological impact and as a form of clinical intervention. A mindfulness based approach has earned increasing respect in medicine, for certain treatments and prevention. There is a huge and ever growing base of evidence confirming the benefits from scientific studies with positive outcomes.

Mindfulness has been offered as a complementary treatment for those suffering a variety of ailments including chronic pain through mindfulness based stress reduction (MBSR), mindfulness based cognitive therapy (MBCT) and more. Mindfulness is also offered as continuous help to people having suffered certain difficult conditions to prevent their relapse and maintain health.

Mindfulness is simply available for anyone who wants to maintain a healthy life.

CHAPTER 2

mindfulness through meditation

2.1. How To Progress

We develop mindfulness in two ways:
1. through meditation, a formal practice of mindfulness.
2. through ordinary daily activities.

For downloadable audio tracks go to: **www.thestrongestyou.net/m-audio** and follow instructions.

Mindfulness can be done in the home without professional help but there are professional services available for those who wish to use them. Like many health related practices mindfulness needs commitment. Many people will start with enthusiasm and quickly give up, real benefits will only come about with regular practise.

Silent meditation is exactly what it says: Being quiet and attend to the mind and body.

Setting the starting time is crucial. We should begin by setting realistic goals and gradually build time. We want to be easy about this and learn to tolerate "doing nothing". It might be completely new and strange when we are told that meditation is just quiet sitting and doing nothing. As a matter of fact, this is one of the hardest tasks. We are so much used to being busy in the mind and restless in the body that we never think it can be otherwise.

Here is a noteworthy benefit of learning to meditate:

In meditation we learn to give a break to the mind and body. Through meditation we can revitalize and recharge.

Despite understanding the benefits of meditation there is still a group of people resistant to meditate. These people just can't do it and only the thought of being still and doing nothing makes them anxious. They can immediately lose interest in meditation or mindfulness.

2.1.1. Ability To Relax

Some people might be discouraged when they are told to silently attend to their mind and body because they just can't stop thinking, quietness is overwhelming, and they are restless. We should understand that silence and doing nothing can be disturbing when people are anxious, depressed, ruminative, or chronically stressed. Also people coping with challenging health conditions or taking some medication might struggle.

Silent meditation might not be good for them but they still can learn mindfulness and benefit from it. They can learn relaxation techniques (reference at the end of this book) and go to silent meditation later.

They also can try:
- sitting in the silence only for a minute a few times daily
- use guided meditation audio tracks if it helps, but they shouldn't force themselves.

2.1.2. Practice Patience

Meditation is something not to be rushed. The ability to meditate is a gradual development of a new skill. As with any other skill we create it through regular practise. When we develop this skill we find comfort and enjoy meditating. Before this happens we have to allow patience. Imagine that we are learning to read in a new language; firstly we learn the alphabet, the sounds of letters, then simple words and lastly read sentences before reading books and understanding what we read. We don't expect much at the beginning when learning meditation.

The goal of silent meditation is to:

Sit silently for a dedicated period of time with closed eyes and in a private place and attend to thoughts and feelings.

2.2. Set the Routine

Remember meditation is a skill and it develops as any other skill through practise. Nobody learns meditation through reading about it. We learn through practising. We develop a routine after clarifying time and place.

Generally five minutes is a good starting point to meditate. If we can manage five minutes twice daily we have made a great start. It's better to do a few minutes in the morning and a few minute in the afternoon. This way we think about mindfulness more often and we are more aware of our target. If we decide to practise in 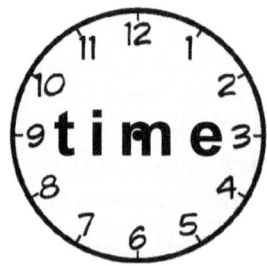 the morning, just after waking up and before starting a day, we must allow enough time; set the alarm at least ten minutes earlier and follow through.

The best time to meditate is early morning when nature and people are waking and beginning the day but if this is not an option practise at a best time.

If we think our schedule is too tight maybe we should look closely how efficiently we use time. Perhaps we find some time reserves when we put few thoughts into efficient time management. We have to put effort in finding time if we want to learn something new. Even when people say they don't have time it still doesn't mean they can't find an extra five to ten minutes daily. Planning is also very important and helpful: Schedule daily meditation at least six to seven days in advance.

We tend to succeed when we schedule and follow through on our planning.

There is no fixed time to developing meditation skills. Some people are very responsive and can move fast to meditations with no time limit. Others need a slower initial pace and steady practise. We should always stay sensible and respond to our feelings to find comfort and our own way of practising.

2.3. Place

There is no strictly advised place where to practice. The best routine builds when we choose a place we can use regularly. Ideally we want to be in a quiet place, undisturbed and allowing ourselves to sit comfortably with closed eyes. It's always better to be alone in a room or be with other meditating people.

We should minimize distractions: turn off the telephone and mobile devices, close doors and let others know we wish not to be disturbed. Some people may prefer dim light, closed curtains or burning candles to deepen their experience. We should avoid practising when we are too tired, after heavy meals or after drinking alcohol.

To monitor time we keep a clock in sight but never set an alarm. To finish gently open the eyes, check the time and gently end or continue to meet the time target.

At times we have to be flexible and when unexpected tasks come we try to fit meditation alternatively between tasks. We can even practise in the car, park the car and meditate prior setting out on a journey. We can meditate during lunch time at parks, prior commuting to or from work, after coming from work, before doing chores or at any other time.

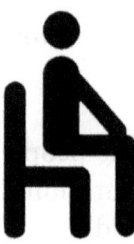 Some people prefer meditating while sitting on the floor in the yoga easy sitting pose: with crossed legs, straight spine, hands rested on the thighs and palms facing up. Other people prefer straight and comfortable sitting on a chair with feet flat on the floor, hands rested on the thighs, back relaxed and straight.

We should assume a relaxed position, gently roll the shoulder to open the chest. We want to be comfortable in sitting when lightly closing the eyes.

2.4. How to Start

The easiest start is to follow the downloadable audio track # 1, but that wouldn't be silent meditation; it would be guided meditation. There is nothing wrong with it and applying previous information we can develop meditation skill through guided meditation. We can do it now but eventually we should experience silent meditation and try it on our own.

When sitting in a comfortable and relaxed position we focus on breathing and bring attention inwardly: into our sensation and the mind. Bringing attention to breathing is important at this stage. Especially when we are new to mediation or when noticing thoughts we redirect attention to breathing. The breath is an anchor helping us not to engage in other thoughts.

We aim just to sit and be distracted as little as possible by thoughts or body; allowing thoughts to come and go, just noticing what happens within us and with our body. We don't try to stop thinking or push thoughts away. Let them come and go and attend to breathing. We want to find comfort in the moment and as thoughts come we redirect attention to breathing, not thinking about past or future. We might need to repeat this many times, over and over.

To finish we open eyes to check the time and gently end. Often the body and mind signal when to end. Meditation shouldn't be rushed so we must allow time and return to our normal tasks.

2.4.1. General Rules

1. Spend a minimum of five minutes daily.
2. Practise daily.
3. Commit to the goal.
4. Take it easy.
5. Regularity is critical.
6. Maintain the focus and mindset to allow learning.
7. Don't rush.
8. Keep a positive attitude.
9. Trust and personalize the statement "I can learn mindfulness".
10. Don't allow giving up.
11. Whatever gets in the way, deal with it.

2.4.2. A Few Tips

An ultimate goal is to silently sit in peace while finding comfort and joy in it. When we relax easily and meet our initial time target only then can we extend the time. The indicator that we are ready to stretch the time is focus and joy. Effortless, non-judgemental sitting, letting thoughts come and go, enjoying the stillness and silence are the signs that we are ready to meditate for a longer time.

Every individual will respond differently and we must wisely choose the length of time that works for us. Consistency is crucial and we should never give up. Even if we skip a practice we return to our previous routine to start again or continue wherever we had finished. We don't want to feel bad about this practice, blame ourselves or be angry when we fail. We rather want to keep a positive attitude and be kind to ourselves in difficulties.

Optionally it may be useful when we take written notes about experiences during meditation: describe how we feel, what thoughts we have, record time and the progress.

PART TWO
MINDFULNESS IN STAGES

3. 1. Aspects of Mindfulness

So far we have focused on meditation. The following chapters explain why and how to practise mindfulness in contemporary life through the application of different aspects of mindfulness. This part explores curiosity, awareness, focus, acceptance, compassion and kindness. There is no strict time for how long we should adopt them. If we can manage to exercise each for at least a week we have made a great attempt. Ultimately we want to change attitude through practising meditation and all aspects of mindfulness.

3.2. Why Is Curiosity Important

Curiosity is an important aspect of mindfulness. There are many activities we do daily without noticing or that we do automatically. When we are curious about the things we do, we engage them. We must bring attention to a present moment when we are curious. Looking at the things with a desire to know deepens our experience. We want to become more interested in the mundane things we do and that other people do. Being curious is to look at the things with interest. We want to use our energy and try to see things in a new light, by looking at them with curiosity and attention.

The ultimate experience is to recognize the magic that is all around us and within us.

3.3. What To Do

Through childhood we have an inherent and insatiable curiosity but for whatever reason, as we grow, this intense curiosity stops. We want to re-introduce curiosity into ordinary daily life to re-discover the charming world. Explore the notion of doing things by noticing their impact. Remember when children ask never-ending questions about how the things work or why people do what they do, when we teach children to understand cause and effect. For this practice we use normal daily activities such as driving, walking, eating, reading, writing.... you name it.

3.4. How To Do It

In formal mindfulness we become curious about breathing, the most essential things we do daily. Breathing is used as an object of our curiosity. We sit in a quiet place with closed eyes and just breathe. Our attention may wander when doing this. That's when we bring attention back to breathing. Breathing is an anchor and is accessible anytime when we lose focus. We become curious about the breath again and again. We might repeat it over as many times as our attention is lost. Curiosity in breathing is to notice what impact the breathing has on the body: what temperature the air has when entering the body and leaving the body, what sensation we feel when breathing, how we feel when focused on breathing, how it impacts on the chest or stomach. We don't have to breathe in any different or particular way. We just breathe normally and become interested in the breath. This practice can take between five to ten minutes.

3.5. Examples How to Enhance Curiosity

We bring curiosity into anything we do however trivial it might be. Similarly to children we can ask any of the central questions: Why? What? How? Who? When? We want to redirect attention from mental chatter, when we are mentally detached from the present moment.

Being interested in what we do takes a conscious effort but it is very beneficial, especially when we notice that we are not fully attending to our current task whatever we do. This is when we should ask the questions of curiosity and start paying attention to what we do.

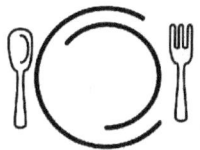 Make eating an exclusive activity meaning you don't do it along with any other activity. Don't read, watch T.V., talk on the phone, walk or play games. Just eat. While eating try to be curious and try to answer questions: What exactly are you eating? How does it taste in your mouth? What benefits does your body get from it? Who made the food? What ingredients did they use? Where did the ingredients come from? How did they make this meal? Could you make it? Be creative and ask a variety of questions.

If you find your attention wondering to other thoughts don't engage them, let them come and go and redirect attention back to eating.

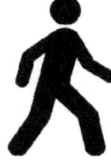 Pay attention to your body and surroundings. Ask questions: How do your feet feel when you are walking? How do your hips feel? What do you do with your arms when walking? What and where in the body you feel impact of walking? Do you feel any tension in the body? How do your clothes feel? What do you see when you walk? What streets do you pass? What natural surroundings can you observe? Can you see trees, flowers, birds, animals, other people? What is the weather like? How does the air feel? How does your breath change when you walk fast or slow? What do you see on the streets? Can you recognize the places or people? Be creative and ask a variety of other questions.

If you find your attention wondering to other thoughts don't engage them, let them come and go and redirect attention back to walking.

CHAPTER 4

awareness

4.1. Why Do We Increase Awareness?

Mindfulness is a form of awareness that rises through paying attention moment to moment and non-judgemental acknowledgement. It is about knowing what is on our mind, what happens in our body and feelings. Awareness as an essential aspect of mindfulness and if we are not sufficiently aware we can't actively influence beneficial change.

In this stage of mindfulness we try to build the ability to attend to our own thoughts, mental chatter, feelings and actions. In childhood we were naturally aware but these days we might lack this awareness, however we can re-develop this skill. Whether we are aware or not, everything that happens in our inner world creates our experiences. What we think and feel affects our actions and choices.

The reason why we want to develop awareness is to deepen the connection with the present moment and current experience.

Once we increase awareness we create a profound understanding of ourselves then consequently, if we wish, we can improve our experience and make it more pleasant.

4.2. What To Do

Simply building awareness is to observe and acknowledge. It is to bring the focus to our own inner experience; to our thoughts, feelings and emotions. We try to describe and identify our experiences in words. We pay attention to how what happens around us impacts on our feelings and thinking. This is something we typically don't exercise. However, if we want to develop mindfulness we should do it. Our thoughts, emotions and feelings are always involved in whatever we do. We might be engaged in thinking that is not necessary and this can make our experience worse.

To develop awareness we:
- use mundane activities and trivial things.
- pay attention to how other people influence our thinking and feelings.
- recognize what in the world around us affects us positively or negatively.
- pay attention to our mind's chatter and self-talks.
- silently meditate.

We practise to recognize our own thinking, mental chatter, internal communication which is normal. It can be in a form of planning, solving problems, thinking about the past or future, about oneself or others, dwelling in the mind on something or someone. We pay attention when doing mindless jobs and chores and we try to notice what we think about and how we think when we do them. We try to non-judgementally acknowledge what impact other people have on us and we gradually start noticing how other activities influence our thinking and feelings.

4.3. How To Do It

Continue silent meditations for about ten or more minutes. While sitting in a quiet place we bring attention to our body. We gently scan the body from the top of the head to the soles of the feet. We hold attention on each body part in turn for a few moments. Focus on how each part feels, if there is tension or relaxation. We practise only awareness and quietly try to notice what happens in the body. If we become judgemental, gently return attention to the bodily sensation.

Exercising awareness can be done through a variety of activities we do daily such as getting ready for work, eating, driving, dropping off children at school, helping others, meeting people, talking to people, talking on the phone, cooking, shopping, watching T.V., listening to the radio, and so on.

We can exercise awareness throughout any activity. As many times as we can we try to acknowledge what we think, how we feel in the body and what emotions we experience. In the mind we try to describe how a certain activity or a person impacts us.

Because this is something new we might need reminders to be alert and not forget doing it. Over time it becomes more automatic. A helpful reminder can be a short written note or we might keep a little pebble in a pocket and each time we touch it, it reminds us. Some people use a message on their mobile devices such as "Notice the inner world". They are gentle reminders to be aware of what's going on within us.

To develop awareness we must remember it from the moment we get up in the morning; we try to catch our feelings and thoughts. We don't explain or judge, we just acknowledge them. Our goal is not to change or halt something. We might be in a hurry as any other morning, perhaps rushing children and ourselves. We might be relaxed and positive when expecting something good. We acknowledge and keep doing as we always do but we should at the same time be aware of how we feel and what we think.

It might be something like: I feel edgy. I am thinking about cooking. I am hesitant. I am frustrated. I am rehearsing for the meeting. I have a headache. My daughter drives me crazy when she is too slow. I am not listening what he said. I am frustrated. I am thinking about the last argument. I am angry because he doesn't want to do what I want him to do.

CHAPTER 5

acceptance

5.1. Why Do We Exercise Acceptance

Acceptance is mental agreement with the present state, with what can't be changed now and might be different in the future. We exercise acceptance to develop mindfulness. Acceptance is the ability to create peace in the mind and consequently it decreases unnecessary stress levels.

Some people reject acceptance because they don't really understand the benefits. Other people might think acceptance is approving something unwanted and acceptance is about giving up. These negative attitudes are not true. Acceptance is making peace with what currently can't be changed. There is no approval or rejection in acceptance. Acceptance is simply to acknowledge something "as it is".

For whatever reason we might try to fight against something that is not in our control. There might be natural limits in ordinary life that we fail to accept. We feel worse when railing against unwanted consequences and limitations. Actions or decisions of other people can be frustrating but we are not in charge of them.

The Buddhists say, "If there is no solution to a problem, there is no problem". Indeed, if we can't resolve something today, we should accept it as it is today. Maybe tomorrow we will be wiser, a situation might improve or we might find a solution. If we can't do anything with something we can't control we should accept it. Acceptance is a necessary aspect of mindfulness.

> Acceptance is actually having the strength to stop fighting limited reality.

5.2. What To Do

This practice can be sometimes difficult to start. We might think that when we accept that which we don't like, it would make circumstances worse. We should remember that we are accepting "as it is today". We are not "locking" a situation or limits, in acceptance we also acknowledge that circumstances can change and improve in the future.

During this stage of developing mindfulness we intentionally accept the limits of our small world. Perhaps, we don't like that the world is full of contradictions, restrictions or conflicts, or that we can't do what other people can do. To accept we must consciously remember that the world and people are not perfect and we all make mistakes. Accepting them should be normal.

We should exercise thinking in terms that current reality doesn't last and what wasn't done today, can be done tomorrow. Exercising acceptance is very important because in the previous stage we developed awareness and now we might more often notice the things we don't like, that we didn't notice before.

Similarly as when practising awareness we learn acceptance through:

- meditation.
- accepting the everyday things we do.
- accepting the things we sometimes have to do but would prefer not to.
- accepting the things other people do that we don't like but can't change.

The important areas where we exercise acceptance are actions and decisions of people including ourselves. Actions of any person, children, siblings, friends, co-workers, bosses, teachers, politicians, journalists, etc. can be something we might struggle to non-judgementally accept. Daily there are almost unlimited opportunities to exercise acceptance.

5.3. How To Do It

To improve acceptance through meditation can be done in two ways. One way is just sitting in a quiet place for ten to fifteen minutes. Our goal is to accept whatever happens within us and around us. We intentionally accept thoughts, sounds, feelings, sensation, and even if we feel pain or discomfort we try to non-judgementally accept it.

The other way of doing it is that we select an issue or a person we might have difficulties to accept. We bring this into our awareness when we meditate and intentionally try to accept. When feeling mental rejection we allow good thoughts and remember that by accepting we help ourselves. We can practice this for five to ten minutes.

While practising acceptance in ordinary life we distinguish feelings from facts. For example we might feel angry with a child who made a mess of their homework. We distinguish feelings, expand our view and re-evaluate our perception. We acknowledge our feelings and thoughts then we consciously change how we think about it. We accept by thinking differently. We might acknowledge that the child was in hurry and stressed, or that they made a mistake. Maybe it was an accident. We consider the good sides such as a child's attempt to do their homework. This evaluation helps us to find peace of mind and accept the mess the child made. Remember, we don't approve it we simply non-judgementally recognize the facts.

There are plenty of situations we encounter daily that give us opportunity to practise: waiting in a queue, having additional work assigned by a boss, being trapped in a traffic jam, missing a train, losing keys, arriving late, our child failing a test, reading the news about a politician we don't agree with, having financial difficulties, having a heated argument with parents, etc. The list of situations we might struggle to accept is endless.

We also deliberately exercise acceptance of ourselves. We might make mistakes, wrong decisions, or even we might be too critical about our appearance or limits. When we notice that we are critical and judgmental we instantly exercise acceptance. "It is as it is" is our new personal statement we wish to identify with. To enhance acceptance we must always base our judgement on facts rather than feelings.

CHAPTER 6

focus

6.1. Why Do We Need To Change Focus

We might be surprised how therapeutic a change of focus can be. People who focus on the negative and on the things they miss can easily become miserable. We might experience self-induced negativity and increase the stress levels just because we wrongly focus. We can't be mindful without controlling focus, without emphasizing the things that we influence and the things that positively impact on our ordinary life.

We should know that we increase efficiency when we just redirect focus. When focused on the things that matter we learn to respond differently to life and people.

6.2. What To Do

Focus involves two aspects, our thoughts and our feelings. These are two characteristics we can be in charge of. We choose where we put our thoughts and consequently we affect how we feel. When focused on misery we choose to feel bad. When focus on good aspects we choose to improve our feelings. Daily we deal with a range of matters we have to resolve and make choices. Our focus determines if we make a situation worse by pondering on something unnecessary and wasteful. By just a slight redirection of focus on what can be done and how it can be done we empower ourselves.

Rather than thinking about stress or limits we exercise our own actions. We might being focused just on problems by themselves instead of focusing on how to resolve them. Similarly to acceptance we focus on the things we impact or control. Sometimes we can't stop or remove something from life but we can change focus to modify how we regard them.

Wrong focus can cause problems to grow. When practising focus we always consider our mental chatter. With awareness and acceptance we intentionally practise where we target our thoughts and feelings. There are daily activities and occurrences that can be sources of additional hardship because we don't deal with them. Focusing on solving problems, being positive and what matters is vital in ordinary life.

An important part of improving focus is also multitasking. Deepak Chopra, an American author and speaker one time said, "Multi-tasking is one of the things we become worse at, the more we practice it". Indeed, we might think multitasking improves our efficiency but the opposite is the truth. When multitasking our focus is distraught. We don't pay full attention to any of the tasks. We do them half-heartedly.

Multitasking is not always a bad thing and we easily can do simple multitasking such as walking and talking. Complex multitasking, however, is a problem. Examples of complex multitasking: driving a car and talking on the phone, sending an e-mail and talking to a friend, writing a text messages and talking to someone in person. Clearly we can't do them at the same time with full attention. We briefly switch attention from one task to the other, back and forth. This decreases our performance and increases stress levels.

Complex multitasking makes us worse at what we are doing.

6.3. How To Do It

At this stage we should be getting better in prioritizing and whenever experiencing distracted focus we should recognize it. We are better in redirecting attention and maintaining a calmer mind. As we continue meditating, directing the focus to breathing and sitting in quietness for about ten minutes, we improve our focus.

As our life can be more stressful some days we should try practising to intentionally reduce stress and distracting thoughts. We can do this practice: While sitting, stretch the arm, hold the thumb up, and fix the sight and full focus on it. As we breathe we hold the sight and try to notice every little detail of the thumb. We let the thumb occupy our mind and don't allow thinking about anything else. If any thoughts disturb our attention we gently close the eyes for a few seconds, then open the eyes and try it again, mindfully observe the thumb. This practice can take between three to five minutes.

We want to decrease doing complex activities in a rush or quickly switching attention from one to other. We want to do them mindfully and efficiently focus on one task at the time. We complete it and then we do the next one. Whenever we realise that we are multitasking, we should stop and redirect focus to only one task. This increases our performance and decreases stress.

Being mindfully focused means we stop rushing through chores or daily actions. We can practice focus in any mundane activity we daily make. We exercise focus along with acceptance and increased awareness.

Development of mindfulness includes focus on resolving, improving and progressing. Exercising focus means to concentrate attention on what can be improved and we do it.

For instance if we are dealing with financial challenges we might be stressed and our mind might be pondering on wrong decisions made in the past, blaming ourselves or others, or any other wasteful thinking. When exercising mindfulness we focus and ask, "What can I do to improve it?" In this case we would focus on how to get finances under control. We might need to create a budget we can stick to, identify expenses that can be decreased, find a financial advisor to help us, or have a family meeting to get everyone on board.

Another example might be when we are frustrated with our partner, we mindfully focus on our expectations and how our partner is or is not able to meet them. We might find problems with our standards, accept limitations and try to non-judgementally understand what, whom and how contribute to a problem.

7.1. What Is Mindful Communication?

Relationships can in one way or another powerfully impact on our life experience. Fruitful relationships improve overall wellbeing and happiness. They offer comfort and intensify security. When we become mindful we realize that we need balanced relationships. The crucial part of relationships is communication.

Not everyone is good in self-expression and mindfulness is a great helper to develop effective self-expression. Sometime we might have difficulties to say what we think, or to say no when we are asked to do something. We might think rejecting someone's requests or additional tasks would be wrong. Mindfulness can help in making this become easier. Through mindful communication we learn to express ourselves in a respectful way which strengthens our position.

Other aspect of communication is listening. Recently more studies suggest that people are become worse listeners than ever. Partially we can blame multitasking and high stress levels. Often we not only fail to listen but we also struggle to non-judgementally respond. When we practice mindful communication we bring full attention to a conversation and listen.

Mindfulness in communication improves relationships. Rather than being a non-constructive critic we become a conscious listener and positively contribute to a relationship. Mindful communication helps in staying grounded and recognizing limits that might negatively impact on relationships.

Through mindful communication we better understand personal accountability, how we and others contribute to a relationship.

7.2. What To Do

How many times does it happen that we talk to someone, agree on something and later we can't remember what was said? In mindful communication this doesn't happen because we exercise both skills, listening and expression.

We shouldn't use conversations as a chance to prove our own agenda. Rather we should converse and listen what the other person has to say. Before we express our own opinion we should ensure that we listen to the other party. We practice interactive communication which means we ensure that we understand what the other person means.

Sometimes we make statements based on our assumptions, without really getting the other party's point and this we want to change. In this stage of development of mindfulness we allow others to speak while avoiding our own pre-emptive or hasty words. We consciously select how and what we say. We think before we speak and avoid making situations less transparent or more tense.

We might habitually use a certain tone of voice, ways of speaking or using words that can negatively affect others or us. We exercise confident and considerate communication.

7.3. How To Do It

Practising mindful communication in daily life shouldn't be difficult. Listening to the other parties is important and we might frequently fail to do it. The new habit we want to develop is taking time, paying attention, not rushing with our opinions or judgements. As we already practise being in the present moment which includes attending to the words of others, we are halfway towards mindful communication.

In formal practise we can continue silent meditation or we can meditate on a phrase "I am a good listener and communicator". In this form of focused meditation we memorize these words and while sitting in a quiet place we play with them in the mind. They might trigger a variety of feelings or bodily sensation which we don't avoid. The goal is to let the mind be occupied by these words. We might notice other thoughts but don't engage them. Just gently redirect attention to the selected words, we might do it many times over and over. This meditation can take ten to fifteen minutes.

There are plenty of situations when we might forget to pay attention to our children, people talking to us on the street or at work. The same way as we attend to our feelings and thoughts we should also practise attending to communication and other people.

Any time we catch ourselves not listening to the other person we gently return attention to them. We can use confirmation phrases to reassure that we get the correct message. Also we gently push ourselves to express ourselves clearly and respectfully, especially when we don't agree with the other party. Staying quiet is not always a bad thing, contrary it is wise to allow time and not to rush or verbally hurt others.

CHAPTER 8
compassion

8.1. Why Do We Learn Compassion?

At this stage of mindfulness we try to practice compassion and self-compassion.

There are some people who might think of compassion as something related to religion. As a matter of fact compassion is a beautiful human quality we frequently overlook. Compassion is a strong antidote to negativity and criticism.

We can all experience situations that trigger us to act for self-protection or to protect people we care about; we might feel an imaginative or real threat. At other times we are driven by excitement or enthusiasm that can developed into attachment. In both cases our flexible thinking is diminished, and we disregard what truly matters to us. We might create attachment and exhibit undesirable behaviour.

When thinking about people we love and their suffering we can be compassionate but when thinking about ourselves it is much harder. Even when we suffer through many causes we become more harsh and self-critical and tend to be emotionally reactive. Self-criticism triggers stress and rejection but we need to heal and release negativity. We need to recognize the wrongful and then put energy to improve, not beating ourselves up for wrong doing. For these reasons we include compassion in mindfulness. With cultivation of compassion and self-compassion we become more caring and positive.

> Compassion activates safe feelings and prevents overreacting when we might detect false danger or react in response to attachments.

8.2. What To Do

This practice might be difficult but we have to put effort into achieving it. There is no mindfulness without compassion. We are critical because we don't want to fail, make or repeat mistakes and we don't want others to fail or make mistakes. We also want to protect others, or for others to be better, and we might think that criticism is what they need.

We want to criticise less, however well meant. In the practice of compassion we avoid severe judgements and try to bring gentleness. When we make mistake we try self-compassion. To cultivate compassion we intentionally become more caring.

We apply compassion through thoughtfulness, gentleness and savouring. Perhaps we notice that it is difficult to appreciate ourselves or might struggle to acknowledge the good within us. The resistance to self-appreciation reduces with conscious practise. Then the mind and brain by themselves respond and improve. The good thoughts manifest in positive feelings. Our task is to redirect thinking from negativity and give the chance to appreciation and gratefulness.

8.3. How To Do It

Compassion is to bring a loving heart into experience and through meditation we can overcome the resistance to be compassionate. Meditation can be a great opportunity to consciously allow it. It can be as simple as sitting in a quiet place and attend to a word compassion, self-compassion, love, gentleness or caring. When we bring full attention into any of these words for five to ten minutes we start feeling their meaning.

The other way of meditating on compassion can be to quietly whisper the phrase, "I am allowing myself to be compassionate". This simple sentence softly repeated as a broken record, over and over can trigger positive feelings and bodily sensation. This practise helps; particularly when doing it over a period of time we overcome the resistance to be compassionate. Meditation can last between ten to fifteen minutes.

We practice compassion and self-compassion in daily life, in ordinary actions and with variety of people. We try to remember it whenever we deal with mistakes, flaws, disappointments, rejections, betrayals or failures. To exercise compassion we take attention away from what and who we criticise and ask what else we can think. We search for kind thoughts we can bring in an issue. We monitor and halt harsh thinking to decrease judgements of ourselves and others. We avoid negative thinking escalating to conflicts, dismissals or disapprovals.

We practice to be less opinionated to decrease our emotional reactions. This helps us think more clearly. When noticing negative and criticising thoughts we take few deep breaths and ask ourselves: What positivity and kindness do I bring into this? What else can I think to help? How does my negativity make it better? Who do my judgements help to?

There can be many occasions when we forget compassion. We might fail to be compassionate about mistakes of our loved ones, ourselves or even people we don't meet daily. Our task is to apply compassion and gentleness whenever we catch ourselves being harsh, judgemental or critical. For this practice we can use any opportunity in personal life, work or school. We can be compassionate about strangers in need and suffering poorer conditions than our own.

CHAPTER 9

kindness

9.1. Why Kindness?

By including kindness into the development of mindfulness we involve psychological aspects of life and human good qualities to create positive experience for ourselves and other living beings. To some this may be regarded as spirituality in its broadest most secular sense.

Through practising kindness we want to become more respectful towards oneself and others; a person whose priority is to care about people, animals and the planet. We exercise kindness in daily life to make our experiences more pleasant and positive.

When we do something for others we feel better about ourselves and kindness really can make us happier. Emotional warmth that we experience in kindness elevates the level of the "good chemicals" in the brain. They spread good feelings, they relax the body, balance hormonal secretion, reduce inflammation. We can say kindness has a positive impact on the whole body and in this way it protects us.

The most apparent positive impact of kindness is on relationships. Kindness allows connecting people, respecting, tolerating the differences and overall makes people better citizens. In many ways lives of people are interwoven, we indirectly depend on each other. Emotional closeness can make us better team players and co-operators. Kindness can create a ripple effect spreading from our families and friends to our society.

9.2. What To Do

We let kindness be our guide. Sometimes it's not easy, especially when dealing with challenging people or issues. Opening to kindness can be very difficult when experiencing negative emotions or negative attitudes. Our intention is important and we must consciously choose the good intention. We deliberately engage in kind self-talks to bring love and tenderness to our hearts. We recognize that kindness towards ourselves, others, animals, and our shared planet positively influences us.

We can develop attitudes that produce positive feelings. We reflect upon our links to family, friends and community instead of merely pursuing self-centred interests and goals. We open ourselves to view difficult situations as opportunities for growth. We stop fixating and attaching on our expectations, on the negative, and draw the power to create positive results. Kindness in daily life starts in our thinking and manifests through our actions.

9.3. How To Do It

At this time we focus meditation on wellbeing, concerns of loved ones or global concerns. The focused meditation can include variety of issues that deserve to be handled with care and love: lack of forgiveness, too much anger, suffering and hurt, issues of self-esteem, acceptance, sadness, fear, trust, or peace. We can devote meditation to a loving person, strangers who suffer or healing of the planet. During this meditation we can be creative and dedicate it to concerns that need kindness.

Bringing kindness into ordinary life is the intention of this stage. We care about our own wellbeing and the wellbeing of others. At the same time we flourish the qualities we have learned during the previous stages of mindfulness.

We might review our beliefs and priorities to know how much they really enhance good values we care about. When experiencing negative emotions we intentionally attend them with kindness and curiosity. We want to understand them and change, stop aggravating negativity. We exercise trust when the things don't go the way we wish. We embrace creativity to open the mind and heart. We exercise acceptance to reduce our attachments or fixation.

PART THREE
IN SUMMARY

CHAPTER 10
living mindfully

This book plants a seed of mindfulness and we might need to pause, take a few moments to allow mindfulness in our lives. But we have to remember we have to nurture and cultivate mindfulness to let it growing.

Hopefully, we have all discovered the important personal meaning that mindfulness can have. Perhaps grounding, peace, focus, balance, calmness, the ability to engage, improved feelings and relationships, gentleness or letting go off rumination and criticism.

The fruit of mindfulness is our protection. It makes us happier at good times and it provides stability in times of turmoil and difficulties. Through mindfulness we can experience spontaneous awareness, joy and peace found within ourselves and in daily life. We shouldn't focus on mindfulness itself but relax and be less self-conscious. We have tried to establish new approaches to living, new habits and routines to make mindfulness an essential part of our daily experiences.

At times it is difficult to be fully present, to break old habits and stop having thoughts ahead of time. To cope with this we literally tell ourselves, "stop" and mindfully re-attend to the moment. Other times we practise easily and with a little effort.

Sometimes we practise mindfulness for a while and then realize we stopped doing it. We might be consumed by a busy life, halted by obstacles and everything else that happens in life, we might forget mindfulness. This happens to almost everyone. Fortunately we know what to do. We know we have to bring our attention to the present moment and breathe.

Breathe in - breathe out. Try mindfulness again. Do it over and over.

ABOUT THE AUTHOR

Now residing in Yorkshire, England Ivana Straska Szakal, M. A., a successful educator and mental health professional, brings inspiration and her unique style to help others. Writing her books with guided practice was inspired by her clients and personal challenges. Her vast experience encouraged her to develop a unique approach that any person can adopt.

Szakal launched her private practice in Toronto in the year 2008 when she became a member of The Association of Registered Psychotherapists & Mental Health Professionals (O.A.C.C.P.P.), Dalton Associates, Psychological & Counselling Services in Ontario. Shortly after she joined GTA Psychological Services and extended her work from Greater Toronto Area throughout Halton and Waterloo Regions. With the development of distant and online services she has been working with many individuals from all walks of life, both in Canada and around the world.

Szakal's first book "The Strongest You" explains how the automatic mode of the mind can cause a dysfunctional service. It teaches coaching of the mind towards positive transformation. The reader is carried forward while purposefully using Szakal's approach tailored to individual's circumstances.

The book "Mindfulness - Breathe In Breathe Out" uses Szakal's knowledge and experience with mindfulness. In an illustrative way it explains how a modern individual can benefit from mindfulness by following simple guidance with a simple "Why? What? How?" approach. The book educates the reader how to live mindfully to feel happier and more satisfied.

Szakal has been practising mindfulness and meditations for over a decade while having an openness towards new approaches for coping with our sometimes frantic modern life. Her academic qualifications are augmented in certified training and extensive experience in the fields of education, psychotherapy, cognitive and behavioural therapy, mindfulness and mental imagery, all of which enforce and support her coaching credibility.

Szakal has a genuine and endearing personality that brings inspiration to others. Her expressed purpose has always been to help people experience the greatest possible fulfilment in their lives.

RESOURCES

Books:

Chambers, R., Ulbrich, M. (2016). Mindful relationships: Creating genuine connection with ourselves and others. Exisle Publishing.

Doidge, N: (2008). The brain that changes itself. Penguin Books Ltd.

Doidge, N. (2016). The brain's way of healing. Penguin Books Ltd.

Hassed, C., McKenzie, S. (2012). Mindfulness for life. Exisle Publishing, Ltd.

Kabat-Zinn, J. (2005). Coming to our senses: Healing ourselves and the world through mindfulness. Piatkus Books, Ltd.

Kabat-Zinn, J. (2013). Full catastrophe living: Using the wisdom of your body and mind to face stress. Random House Publishing Group.

Neff, K. (2011). Self-compassion: Stop beating yourself up and leave insecurity behind. HarperCollins Publishers Inc.

Szakal, I. S. (2017). The Strongest You. 12 week programme with techniques and audio tracks. Ivana International. England.

Thondap, T. (1998.) The healing power of mind: Simple meditation exercises for health, well-being and enlightenment. Shambala Publications Boston & London.

Websites:
www.feel-good.xyz/
www.ivanaszakal.com
www.thestrongestyou.net/
www.ncbi.nlm.nih.gov/
www.mind.org.uk/
www.nhs.uk/
www.nice.org.uk/
www.sciencedirect.com/
www.self-compassion.org/
www.smilingmind.com.au/
www.themindfulnessinitiative.org/
www.umassmed.edu/

For downloadable audio tracks go to:
www.thestrongestyou.net/m-audio and follow instructions.

www.ingramcontent.com/pod-product-compliance
Lightning Source LLC
Chambersburg PA
CBHW060034040426
42333CB00042B/2442